THE BIRTH OF A CHILD

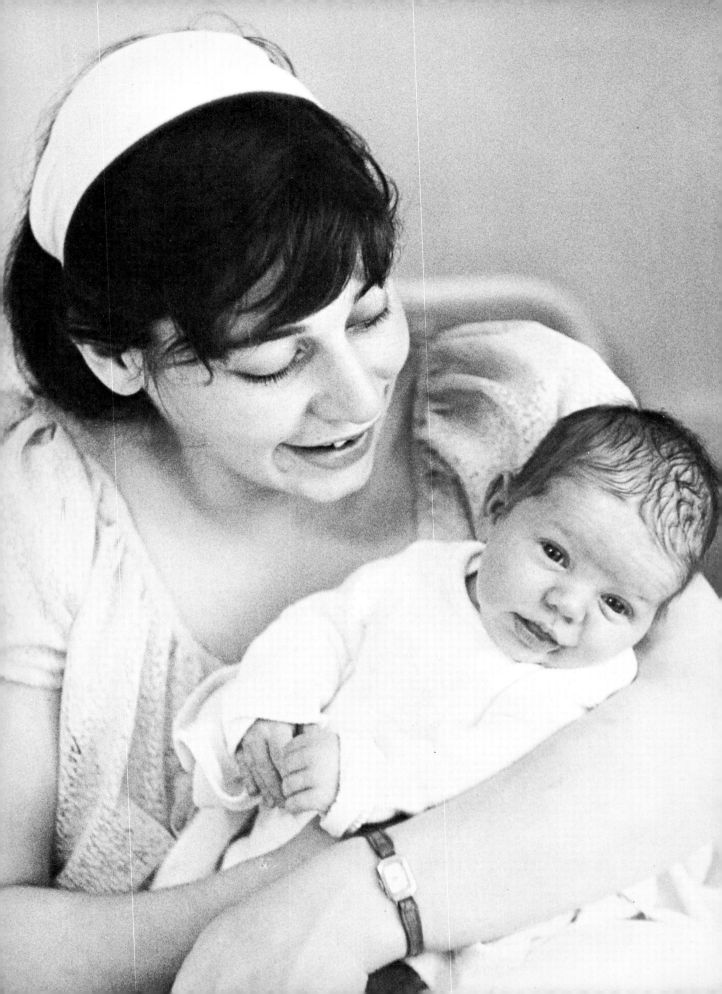

THE BIRTH OF A CHILD

A Doctor's-Eye-View Documentary
of a Child Being Born

Text by ANN DALLY
M.A., M.B.B.S., D.Obst., R.C.O.G.

Photographs by RONALD SWEERING

With a foreword by JOSEPHINE BARNES
M.A., D.M., M.R.C.P., F.R.C.S., F.R.C.O.G.
CONSULTANT OBSTETRICIAN AND GYNAECOLOGIST, CHARING CROSS HOSPITAL
AND THE ELIZABETH GARRETT ANDERSON HOSPITAL, LONDON

With an introduction to the American edition and modification of the text by
ALAN F. GUTTMACHER, M.D.
PROFESSOR EMERITUS, OBSTETRICS AND GYNECOLOGY, THE MOUNT SINAI MEDICAL SCHOOL
VISITING PROFESSOR, OBSTETRICS AND GYNECOLOGY, THE ALBERT EINSTEIN MEDICAL SCHOOL
PRESIDENT, PLANNED PARENTHOOD FEDERATION OF AMERICA, INC.

CROWN PUBLISHERS, INC., NEW YORK

Photographs © 1964, 1969, by Ronald Sweering
Text © 1965, 1969, by Ann Dally
First published in the U.S.A. 1969 by Crown Publishers, Inc.
Originally published in Great Britain as *A Child Is Born*
Library of Congress Catalog Card Number: 77–75062
Manufactured in the United States of America

INTRODUCTION

to the American Edition

BY ALAN F. GUTTMACHER, M.D.*

THE physiology of birth has probably remained unchanged for hundreds of thousands of years. And the process is virtually the same for every mammal, be it a mouse with a 21-day pregnancy terminating in the delivery of several young weighing a few ounces, a woman whose pregnancy lasts 280 days delivering a 7½-pound baby, or a whale with a 730-day gestation ending in a single fetus weighing hundreds of pounds. In each, when the day of birth arrives, the muscular uterus assumes a different and more powerful contraction pattern that creates enough force to propel the fetus inch by inch through the birth canal and into the outside world. In the human, the force of a single labor contraction has been measured at between 35 and 50 millimeters of mercury, differing in intensity from other mammals according to weight, size, and other factors perhaps not so well known.

---

* President, Planned Parenthood Federation of America, Inc.

The human race is distinguished also in another aspect of the birth process. All mammals except the human eat the placenta shortly after parturition; it makes no difference if they are herbivorous like the cow or carnivorous like the lion. How and why this instinct evolved is the content of biological essays. One author believes that it is to remove all traces by sight or smell of the recent birth, since new mothers with helpless offspring are at a great disadvantage against predators. Another suggestion is that the hormone-rich afterbirth contains valuable chemicals to promote lactation and the return of the reproductive organs to normal. Humans notwithstanding, in all primitive societies the placenta is promptly buried with well-established ritual.

Despite such predictable behavior, and the fact that the mechanics of labor itself have remained unchanged throughout the ages, the response and adaptation of animals to the process of birthing have changed. Probably in the not too distant past human females delivered much as the monkey I once observed. With the onset of labor she became restless, walked, and climbed about. As labor progressed, she examined herself repeatedly, placing her fingers within the vagina to feel for the baby. As the head was about to be born, the monkey squatted and attempted to grasp the baby's head, and, when this became possible, extracted the fetus and licked it all over, probably because it tasted delightfully salty from the amniotic fluid that wet its fur. She then put the babe to the breast. The suckling caused further labor contractions, and the mother squatted once again and expelled the placenta, which still remained attached to the baby by its navel cord. The mother climbed about with the baby at the breast, the attached placenta swinging back and forth like a pendulum. After a few minutes she sat on the ground and severed the cord with her teeth an inch or two from the infant's belly button. She then proceeded to devour the afterbirth with apparent relish, licking her fingers.

Since the time of comparison with the monkey, human obstetrical care, as well as customs, has changed materially. In the days of classic Greece and Rome, every proper house had a shallow pit at ground level. When the lady of the house labored, she sat before it upon a birth stool with the center of the seat removed. The midwife stood or crouched in the pit so that her arms were at a comfortable level to accomplish delivery. During the seventeenth century, *le lit du travail,* the labor bed, replaced the birth stool. Previous to the eighteenth century it was deemed improper for male physicians to attend a woman in normal labor; this was the exclusive task of midwives. And if a physician was called to care for an abnormal situation, he was not permitted to observe the birth area, for delicacy demanded that it be covered from his gaze by a "modesty cloth." If any manipulation was required, he carried it out beneath the covering through sense of feel. This was changed by Louis XV. A midwife was good enough to deliver the queen of her seven children, but when it came to the delivery of his favorite mistress the king insisted that a male physician handle the whole case, even though everything was normal. I am not certain, but perhaps the "modesty cloth" was eliminated on the same occasion. Since a king can do no wrong, his subjects copied the royal example.

Man's reaction and adaptation to birth differ not only with the passage of time but also with the location of birth. A normal birth deep in the African bush involves the same physiologic process that it does in a great modern university hospital in the United States, but that is where similarity ends. Even birth in a fine Dutch hospital differs in many details from delivery in an equivalent institution in this country. The fascinating and extraordinary photographs that illustrate *The Birth of a Child* demonstrate this. The absence of caps and masks on delivery-room personnel, the visit of a child to his mother while in labor, the strange, one-eared stethoscope that the physician uses, and incomplete shaving of the birth area depict some of the minor differences between obstetrics in Holland and in our own country. To be sure, there are more similarities than differences. It is apparent that the mother is successfully experiencing natural childbirth in the manner many do in our own maternities. The doctor's maneuvers to deliver the head without damage to the mother's tissues and his handling of the umbilical cord beside the baby's head are what we practice and teach American medical students. As a fellow "stork" of long experience I admire the technique displayed when the doctor removes mucus from the baby's mouth and throat as well as the care employed when he examines the afterbirth to make sure none remains behind.

A mother who delivers a baby either in Holland or in the United States in 1969 is a fortunate woman because never in world history have pregnancy and birth been so safe for both. Having begun obstetrical training in 1925, and practice in 1929, I have been a part of this happy revolution. In the mid-twenties in the United States, over 700 women died for each 100,000 babies born; by 1940, the number had diminished to 317; in 1950, to 75; and in 1966, the last year for which we have figures, the rate is 29. No doubt it is even slightly lower for 1968. Unfortunately, the unhappy fact still exists that risk from birth is higher among nonwhites than whites in this country. The maternal death rate in 1966 per 100,000 white births was 20 (1 in 5,000) in contrast to 72 per 100,000 (1 in 1,400) for nonwhite births. This discrepancy is probably not due to ethnicity, but to the greater occurrence of poverty among nonwhites, resulting in a higher incidence of malnutrition, poorer home environment, and inferior medical care.

During my professional life of four and a half decades, I have also witnessed improvement in the baby's chances for survival, but not to the same miraculous degree as the mother's. If 1,000 white women carry a pregnancy beyond 28 weeks, that is, do not miscarry, 969 can anticipate that the baby will be born alive and survive the first month of life; for nonwhites the expectation is 946 survivors per 1,000. Both figures are a 50 percent improvement over those of 25 years ago.

The recent improvement in maternal childbirth risk and infant survival in the United States is mirrored by most of the industrialized countries of the world. Actually, the Netherlands and the Scandinavian countries are in first place by a small margin, which is probably due to their relative lack of poverty and slums, as well as their high state of nutrition.

All this proves the adage that there are many ways to skin a cat. In the United States, 97 percent of births occur in hospitals, while in the Netherlands the figure is only 30 percent. In the United States virtually every birth is attended by a physician, while in the Netherlands 35 percent are attended by nurse-midwives. Yet despite these differences, the results are approximately the same.

In addition to pregnancy and birth being safer in 1969 than they were 25 years ago, I think having a baby is more fun. Most of the grim don't's have been removed, and pregnant women can play tennis, ride horseback, or hold a job. Then, too, women feel better. Serious nausea and vomiting are things of the past. Today in America because of the many parents-to-be classes and wide availability of lay literature such as *The Birth of a Child,* mystery, fear, and ignorance about having a baby have been replaced by facts, confidence, and knowledge.

I witnessed the introduction of heavily medicated childbirth into obstetrics in the United States in the late twenties, with patients so deeply sedated and anesthetized that they were the last to know they had become mothers. On many, many occasions, part of my duty as stork was to persuade an incredulous woman several hours after delivery that her labor was over and that the son or daughter was already safely deposited in the nursery. The most convincing method was to guide the patient's hand and let her feel the replacement of her pregnant, mountainous bulge by a newly acquired abdominal valley. Mothers desiring such extensive pain relief are usually disinterested in nursing.

Then, too, such a full pain-relief regimen isolates the patient from her husband and other relatives; as soon as labor is well established and analgesia is begun, the family is dismissed. Many husbands go home or to the nearest bar to be summoned when the stork is in the vicinity of the chimney and about to deposit the bundle of joy.

Thoughtful, intelligent, emotionally mature couples found this unsatisfactory for two reasons. First, the husband was left out of the birth process entirely; he was relegated to the status of a prize bull. Second, though the mother had gone through the discomforts of nine months of pregnancy, when the great moment came she was mentally as disconnected from it as though her head had been disarticulated from her body.

At about this time natural childbirth came into being—the Grantly Dick-Read method in England and the psychoprophylactic technique of the Parisian Lamaze, by way of Russia. There are separate books and courses for parents that describe and teach both, so there is no need to enter into an in-depth analysis of them in this introduction. Suffice it to say that for many couples natural childbirth suits their personal needs brilliantly. The expectant father becomes a person, a potential parent instead of the inseminator. He reads with his wife and frequently attends classes for the expectant couple. In many instances he becomes his wife's lay medical adviser. Usually the husband remains in the labor room with his wife throughout labor, giving her valuable support. In some hospitals, after being gowned and masked, the father is admitted to the delivery room, and witnesses the birth.

During pregnancy the mother is desensitized to the pains and rigors of labor by the removal of fear and ignorance from the birth process and by being taught to relax and to anticipate labor with happiness devoid of anxiety. This understanding, confident attitude reduces the need for drugs so that in many cases throughout labor no pain-relieving analgesic is necessary; in other cases one or two injections of Demerol suffice. In either instance the mother is awake and attends the birth of her own child not only physically but mentally as well. She is likely to watch the actual birth in a properly focused mirror, and will hear her baby's first cry. And if the father is allowed in the delivery room, they will share this moment together.

Then, too, in natural childbirth mothers are more likely to suckle the baby. If there is a "rooming-in" setup at the hospital, a natural-childbirth baby is wide-enough awake to begin demand-feedings within a few hours.

I realize that all women and all couples are not alike, and therefore state with complete conviction that natural childbirth is splendid for some and wretched for others. A frank discussion with one's physician is likely to place the situation in perspective so that proper choice can be made. In either instance, knowledge of the process of birth is a valuable asset, and these revealing, marvelous photographs in *The Birth of a Child* can do much to furnish some of this knowledge.

January 6, 1969

FOREWORD

to the British Edition

BY JOSEPHINE BARNES
M.A., D.M., M.R.C.P., F.R.C.S., F.R.C.O.G.

THIS book is about childbirth, in fact about one particular woman's experience at the birth of her second baby. It is a record of an individual event in the life of a Dutch family.

The publication of this book is a bold venture. There are to my knowledge few books which describe and illustrate normal childbirth in such a realistic way. There is nothing in it to shock or horrify. It presents the birth process for what it is, one of Nature's most astonishing achievements, a miracle repeated so often, yet always new, always different.

Nowadays it is quite common for a father to witness the birth of his child, and many men have shared this great experience with their wives. In this case the husband was not only present during the labour and birth but took the remarkable series of photographs which illustrate this book.

This was in every way a model of what a "normal" birth is; it did not last long; the mother did not suffer excessive discomfort or pain but was well relaxed and confident most of the time. The baby was healthy.

This mother was delivered by a doctor. Remember that this birth took place in Holland where there are certain differences in organisation and technique in the management of childbirth. In Great Britain a normal second birth like this one would most probably be conducted by a midwife and might take place in the patient's own home rather than in hospital. British midwives have an exceptionally good record in the safe management of normal births.

Some points of difference in technique will be noticed by those accustomed to seeing mothers in labour. For example, in this country it is usual to insist that all those attending the mother in labour, including the father, wear masks. The photographs of the mother's private parts show that they have been only partly shaved. Some doctors and midwives do this here, but in most cases the hair is completely removed; this is a matter of individual practice. The mother is generally given an enema to empty and cleanse the lower bowel at the beginning of labour.

In many hospitals, or in her own home, the mother may be given something to inhale during the last part of labour. This may be nitrous oxide ("laughing gas") with air or with oxygen, or Trilene. Some mothers find this a help; others, and especially those who have been carefully prepared during pregnancy, find they do not need this help. Some will even refuse it.

Standards of maternity care have improved so much all over the world that the achievement of normal childbirth should be within the reach of almost every woman. Over 80 percent of births are as normal as this one. For the minority who cannot achieve normal childbirth, there are now safe methods of help which should be made available to all. Preparation for childbirth, good care during pregnancy, safe methods for pain relief when needed, and skill in handling difficult cases all contribute much to the well-being of mother and child.

THE BIRTH OF A CHILD

THE BIRTH OF A CHILD

THE following pages show what happened when a baby was born. The record is probably as typical of normal childbirth as any individual record could be, but it is only the story of how one particular baby was born, not of how all babies are born.

Each baby is different and each labor is different. Although there are certain events that must take place during every birth, they do not always occur in the same way, in the same order, or at the same speed. A baby may take many hours to be born or he may arrive so quickly that he gives scarcely any warning at all. He may be born head first, feet first, bottom first, or face first. The descent and birth of the baby's head may be a slow business lasting for an hour or more (if it lasts longer than this, the birth will probably be hastened by delivering the baby with forceps), or it may happen so quickly that the doctor has no time even to wash his hands before delivering the baby. In Britain a doctor is called only if there are complications; only a minority do normal deliveries.

In this book we have tried to present the birth of a baby as it is, and not in an idealized form. Normal people involved in a normal birth usually find it neither horrific nor disgusting. But it can be rather a shock the first time, and this is true both if you are producing the baby yourself or watching its birth. It is also very hard work for the mother, and "labor" is the right word for it.

Most mothers also find it painful, at least at certain stages. Some women say they feel no pain, but they are a minority. Many people who work with mothers in labor believe that the word "pain" should not be used. Instead they talk about "contractions" or "sensations." But the woman who knows that pain is one of the many sensations that she will probably encounter during her labor is better prepared for it than the woman who expects only vague "contractions" or "sensations." On the whole, I prefer not to use the word "pain" very often, but I have used it sometimes, when it expresses the true sensation most accurately.

No ONE KNOWS why labor starts or why it continues. It is one of the mysteries of life that we do not yet understand. We can start the process of labor artificially, but only if the woman is ready for it. We do not know the exact nature of the nervous and chemical changes that control it.

The expected day of the baby's birth, known as the E.D.C., or Expected Date of Confinement, is calculated as 9 months and 7 days from the first day of the last menstrual period, a total of 280 days or 10 lunar months. But this is purely for convenience. No one can forecast exactly when a baby will be born, and those who appear to do so have simply made a good guess.

If a woman's periods are regular, there is a 75 percent chance that her baby will be born within a week of her Expected Date. One in four of all babies is born earlier or later than this.

At the end of pregnancy the baby usually weighs between 5 and 10 pounds and is about 20 inches long. He usually lies head downward in his mother's womb. The fundus, or top of the uterus or womb, reaches somewhere near her ribs, and this is probably rather uncomfortable.

Inside the uterus the baby floats in his bag of waters, which usually contains two to three pints of a liquid called the "amniotic fluid." His umbilical cord, which is about the same length as himself and contains blood vessels and a protective jelly, runs from his navel to the placenta, or afterbirth. The placenta is rather like a large thick dinner plate, from which, in Latin, it derives its name. It has two surfaces, one, rather rough and ragged, the maternal surface, the one attached to the inner muscle wall of the uterus, and the other, smooth and glistening, the fetal surface, which is covered by closely applied fetal membranes. These membranes rise from the fetal surface and form a strong, two-layered bag of waters that contains the baby and a quart or two of salty, warm amniotic fluid, which surrounds and protects the baby until birth. Blood from the mother in its own thin-walled system circulates through the placenta and comes in close contact in the placenta with the blood of the fetus in its own thin-walled system. The fetal blood is brought to the placenta by the baby's heart, which pumps it into the placenta through the vessels of the umbilical cord. When the two bloods, that of the mother and the baby, come into close contact, waste products from the baby, such as CO_2, lactic acid, and urea, pass over into the mother's bloodstream and are eliminated by her lungs and kidneys. Foodstuffs, such as oxygen, glucose, fats, and proteins, pass from the mother's to the baby's blood. The mother's blood passes through the baby's body through the umbilical cord and the baby's bloodstream; the "building blocks" of the blood are then distributed to its tissues and enable the fetus to grow. The baby's CO_2 passing from the baby's into the mother's blood and the mother's oxygen passing from her blood into the baby's in reality accomplishes precisely what a lung does in postnatal life, that is, the elimination of CO_2 and the acquisition of oxygen. In these terms, the mother breathes for her baby.

Every pregnancy must end in labor (unless it is ended artificially by cesarean section). Labor is the process in which the mother's womb or uterus gradually opens and expels the baby, the bag of waters, and the afterbirth. It does this by a series of strong contractions during which the uterus becomes hard and round.

The uterus has a very special sort of muscle that is not found anywhere else in the body. It is capable of contracting in the special, rhythmical way that is necessary in childbirth. Also, unlike any other muscle, after each contraction it is a little shorter than it was before, even when it is relaxed.

Another unusual feature of the muscle of the uterus is that it is designed to work only a few times in a lifetime. In fact, after the third or fourth baby it tends to become progressively inefficient, and this is one of the reasons why women who have borne many babies require special care during labor.

During the first stage of labor the mouth of the womb or cervix is gradually opening. The mother plays a purely passive role. The second stage of labor is concerned with the expulsion of the baby, and here the mother may play an active part. During the third stage of labor the afterbirth is born. The baby plays a passive role throughout.

As often happens, this mother's labor began slowly. The first signs were regular twinges in her back, due to the contractions of the uterus. Her uterus had been contracting and relaxing all her life, but with pregnancy the contractions become more marked, gaining in intensity as pregnancy advances. Suddenly, the contractions pass from unimportant pregnancy contractions, which cause no pain, to labor contractions that she feels. She knows that the time has come to go to the hospital.

When she arrives at the hospital she is given an admission examination by the intern or resident on duty or her own physician, who makes sure that everything is normal, and assesses how far her labor has progressed.

OCCASIONALLY babies are born in ambulances or while the mother is being wheeled into the hospital, but usually there is plenty of time to do everything slowly. Awaiting her at the hospital is the full record of her pregnancy, so that those who look after her can see what has happened during the previous months. The patient undresses and probably takes a bath. She dresses in a short labor garment, and a nurse comes and shaves her, which is what she is doing in the photograph. The shaving is done for hygienic reasons. Germs flourish in and around hair. In the later photographs you will see that this mother is only half shaved. In most American hospitals all the pubic hair is shaved, and the nurse would wear a mask and a cap. Also, it is customary in the United States to administer an enema. This cleanses the lower bowel, lessening the likelihood of contaminating the birth area by involuntary passage of stool material late in labor.

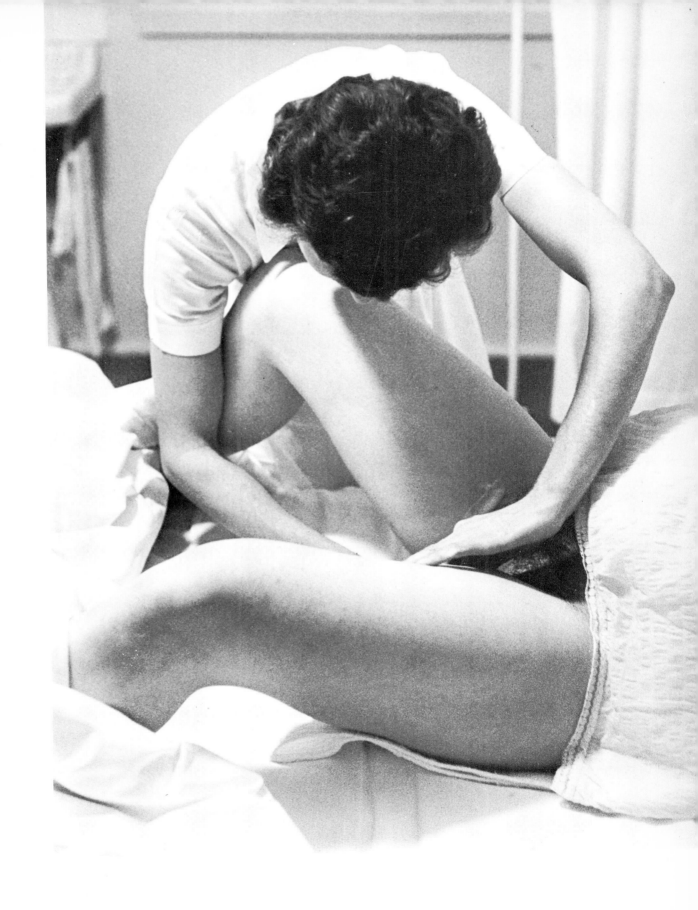

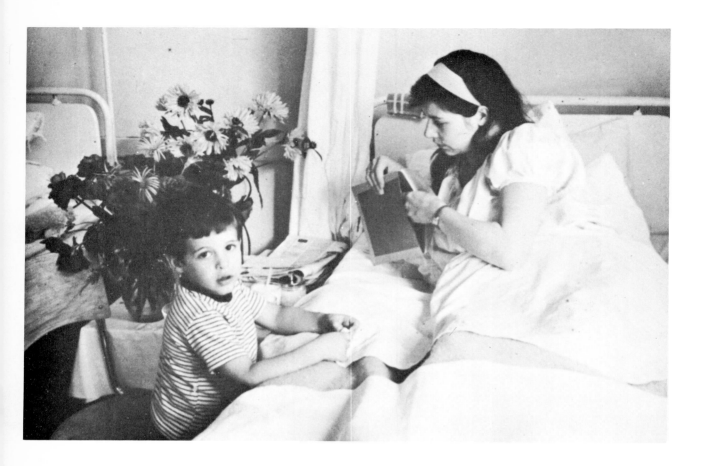

THE MOTHER GETS INTO BED, but unless her waters have already broken she is probably still allowed to walk around. This mother is lucky. She is allowed to see her small son. I do not know of any United States hospital that would allow this. They are not trying to be unpleasant, but so often a child is incubating an infection that he could unwittingly bestow upon his mother or, worse, leave germs behind for the baby as yet unborn.

The first stage of labor is usually the longest. With a first baby it often lasts for 12 hours or more. Even with a second baby it often lasts somewhere between 4 and 12 hours. But this is only a rough guide. It may be much longer or shorter than this.

During the first stage of labor, the mother is supposed to relax as much as possible, especially when she has a pain, and to keep up her strength with adequate nourishment. On the other hand, if it is planned to carry out the delivery under anesthesia, particularly inhalation anesthesia, all fluids or food by mouth may be denied her throughout labor. If the labor is long, she may be hydrated and fed with intravenous glucose.

As LABOR PROGRESSES she feels the need to rest. The contractions are coming more strongly and more frequently, and she wants to concentrate on what is happening. She lies on her bed, relaxing as the contractions come in the way that she has been taught.

Inside her the baby lies quietly in his bag of waters, which has not yet broken. The waters usually break at the end of the first stage of labor when the cervix or mouth of the womb is fully dilated and the baby is ready to be born. But they may break at any time. In about one birth in five, labor actually starts in this way before there have been any pains at all. Once the waters have broken, the mother may be advised to stay in bed in case the cord slips down in front of the baby.

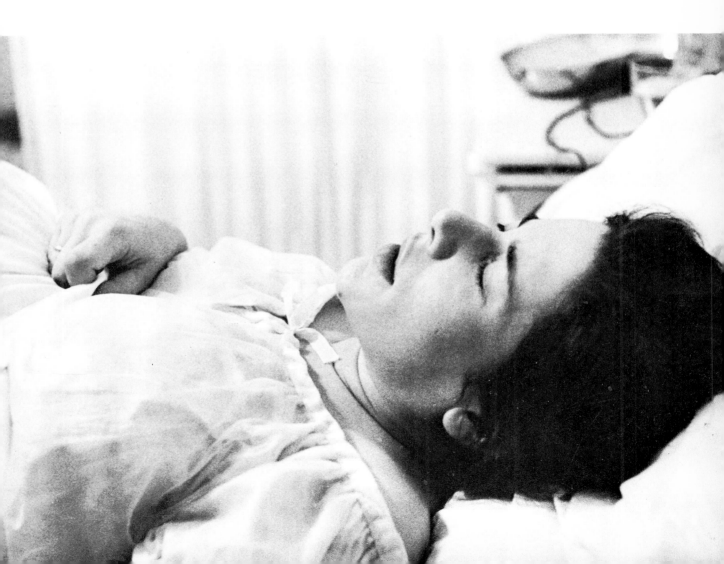

THE DOCTOR COMES to examine her. A woman in labor is examined frequently by a doctor so that complications can be prevented before they arise. The doctor times the pains with his watch, feels her stomach, makes sure that the baby is in the right position, and listens to the baby's heart through a stethoscope. The baby's heart beats much faster than his mother's, about 120 to 140 times a minute. It makes a characteristic sound which the untrained ear finds hard to hear. In Europe, where these excellent pictures were taken, a monaural stethoscope, a simple metal or wooden tube with a large round end, is commonly used to listen to the fetal heart. In the United States, the biaural variety is used or a special fetal scope that differs from an ordinary stethoscope. A fetal scope has a headband and fits over the forehead, not unlike a miner's lamp, which intensifies the sound, through bone as well as air conduction.

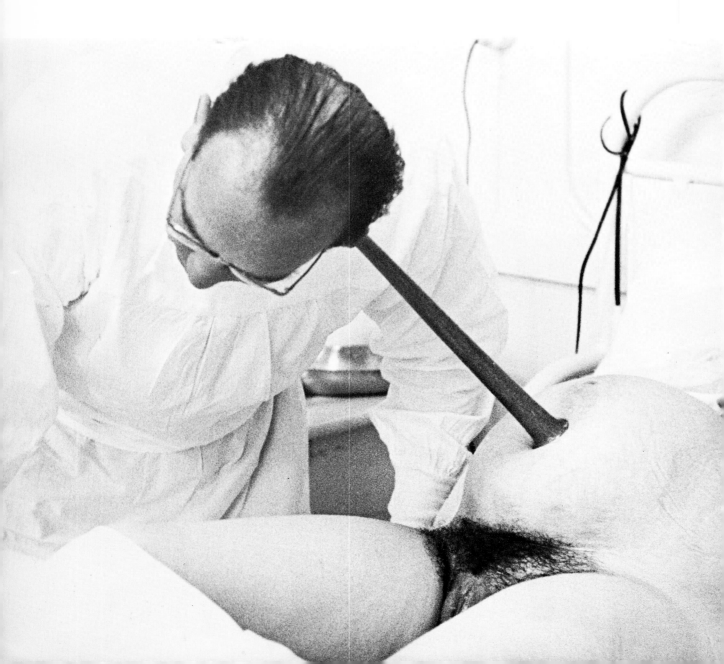

DURING THIS FIRST STAGE of labor the cervix, which is the mouth of the womb, is gradually opening. Neither the mother nor the baby play an active part in this, but fear and nervous tension can delay it. The amount by which the cervix is dilated can be assessed by internal examination, and is measured in centimeters or else in "fingers," according to how many fingers it admits. One Finger dilatation is scarcely anything, and Five Fingers, near the end of the first stage of labor, is called Full Dilatation.

The cervix dilates by a gradual shortening of its muscle fibers. At every contraction the muscle that is the wall of the uterus contracts, and each time it relaxes after a contraction the muscle fibers are left a little shorter than they were before. This shortening of the muscle gradually opens the mouth of the uterus.

The process of dilation is helped if the baby's head is pressed down onto the cervix, which it usually is. The baby's head then fits into the lower segment of the uterus, and at each contraction the muscle fibers are drawn up round it. When the muscle relaxes, a little more of the baby's head appears in the gap made by the dilating cervix.

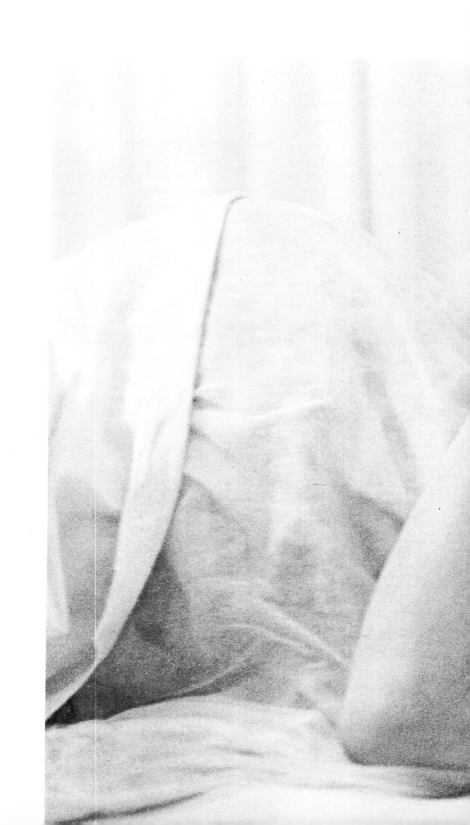

THE MOTHER LIES quietly and is relaxing well. Between contractions she feels comfortable and peaceful and may even sleep. If labor is long, the ability to relax between pains will help enormously. A drug such as pethidine (Demerol), which is often given during the first stage of labor, helps to dull the pain and greatly increases the mother's rest between contractions.

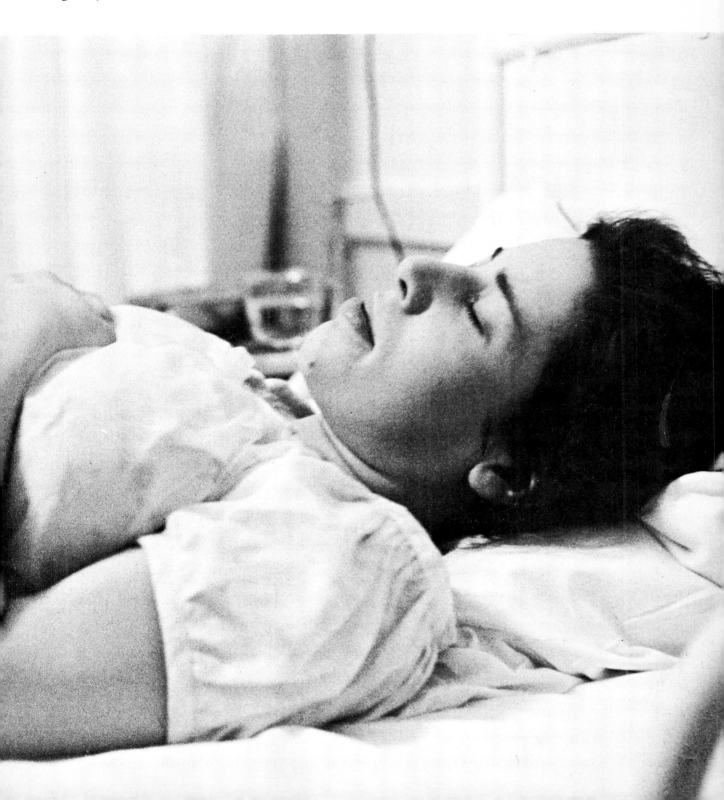

SHE IS AWAKENED by a sensation of a new severity. It takes her by surprise, and she screws up her face.

At this stage the doctor will probably review the situation and perhaps examine the mother internally. If labor is likely to last for some considerable time, the mother may be given a sedative or pain-killing drug.

But this particular mother is far on in her labor, and those last two or three pains, the most severe that she will have to endure, came right at the end of the first stage as the cervix of the uterus became fully dilated. The waters often break at this stage, though by no means always.

At about this time, if not before, she is probably wheeled into the delivery room where her baby will be born.

The mother now feels a new sensation. With every contraction she also feels a desire to push. As soon as it is determined by examination that the neck of the womb is fully open, that is, the cervix is fully dilated, the mother is encouraged to push with every pain.

At this stage of labor the active cooperation of the mother is important. The baby's passage into the world can be greatly helped or hindered by the effectiveness of the mother's pushing. The muscular wall of the womb is itself contracting in efforts to expel the baby, but it will be aided by the proper use of the mother's powerful voluntary muscles, especially the diaphragm and the abdominal wall. The mother is encouraged to take a short breath, hold it, and push down hard, as if expressing a hard stool. In this way the diaphragm is fixed, the muscles of the abdominal wall contract, and a tremendous pressure helps to push the baby in the right direction.

Some women seem to push quite naturally in the correct manner. Others find it difficult and tend to be ineffective, perhaps pushing in the wrong direction or simply lifting themselves up into the air. When the mother knows how to push properly, the baby arrives more quickly.

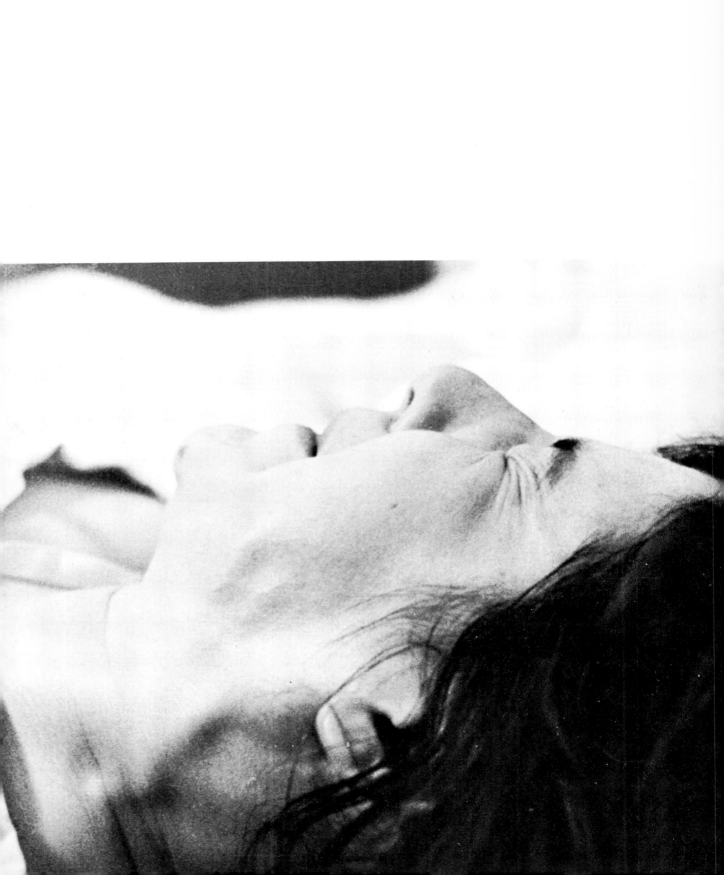

THE MOTHER IS now in the second stage of labor. The cervix of the womb is fully dilated so that the child can pass through. Each time she feels a contraction she bears down forcefully, and the baby inches down a little. Although the contractions are strong, most mothers prefer the second stage to the first stage because they have something positive to do, and pushing with the contraction helps to relieve the pain. Many mothers feel no pain during this stage.

In this way the baby is slowly expelled by the powerful contractions of the mother's womb, with the aid of her own voluntary efforts.

The second stage of labor is often short and easy, particularly with a second baby. If it lasts for more than about an hour, the doctor will probably assist the baby's birth with forceps. But sometimes the second stage is so easy that the mother scarcely has to make any effort at all.

THE ATTENDANTS REALIZE that the patient's labor is progressing well. Since it is a second baby, they know that it probably will not last long now. They send for her doctor. He dresses up in a special sterile gown and puts on sterile rubber gloves. In the United States he would certainly wear a mask and cap, and so would all others in the labor room. This is to avoid risk of transmitting infection to mother or baby. Immediately after the birth, the lining of the birth canal is raw and can easily become infected if proper care is not taken. Until about 1935, puerperal fever killed many women after childbirth. It was caused by a germ called the hemolytic streptococcus, which, through the widespread use of antibiotic drugs, has been virtually eliminated. It was commonly cultured from the throats of well people, carriers, and, not infrequently, from hospital dust; today it is infrequently encountered. Nowadays, puerperal fever

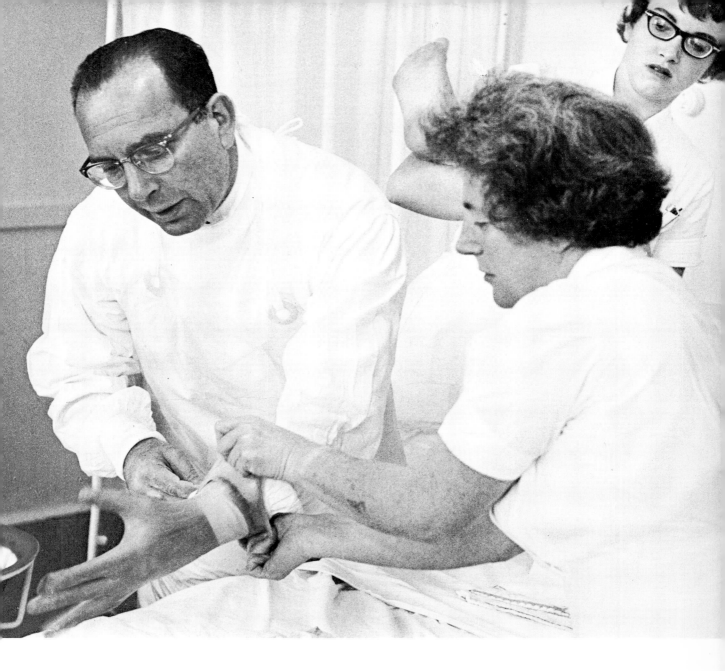

is much rarer and milder, and it is caused by different germs. It can often be cured quickly with antibiotics. Though it is not the menace that it was in former days, every precaution is taken to see that infection does not occur.

Because new babies have had no previous contact with germs, they are also liable to develop infection. Nurses usually wear masks when handling them, particularly in wards and nurseries where many babies are together and infection can spread easily. A mother, who is handling only her own baby, is not usually expected to wear a mask. A baby quickly gets used to his own mother's germs and also to those of his family.

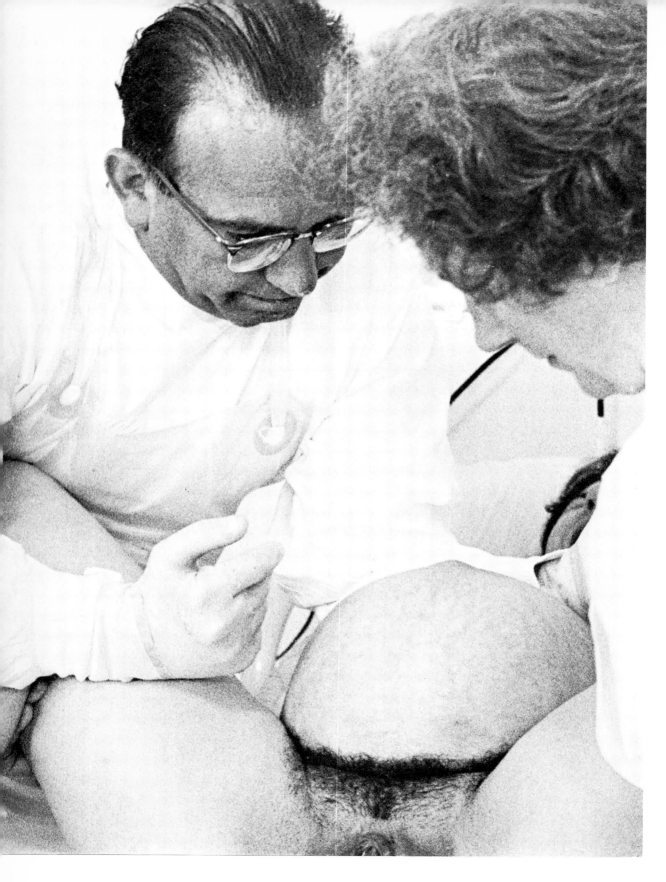

THE DOCTOR AND THE NURSE WAIT for the mother to have a contraction so that they can see what is happening.

WITH THE NEXT CONTRACTION about two inches of the baby's head suddenly come into view. This is an exciting moment. At this stage the mother probably feels discomfort rather than pain, as though she wanted to pass a large stool.

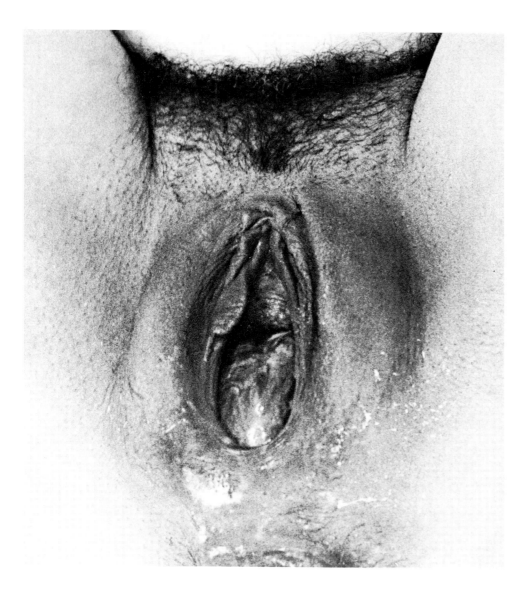

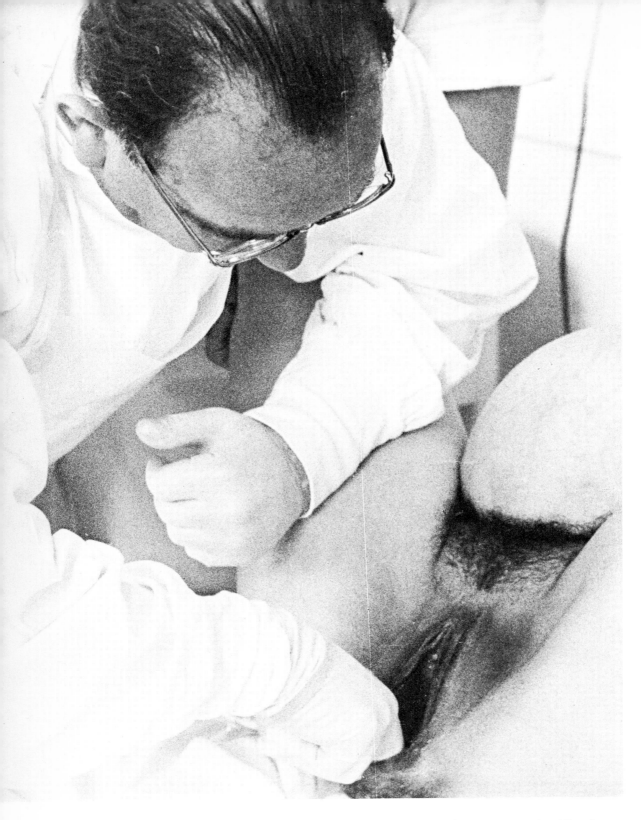

THE PAIN PASSES and the baby's head retracts and disappears again. The doctor gently pulls down the vagina to see how far the head has retreated.

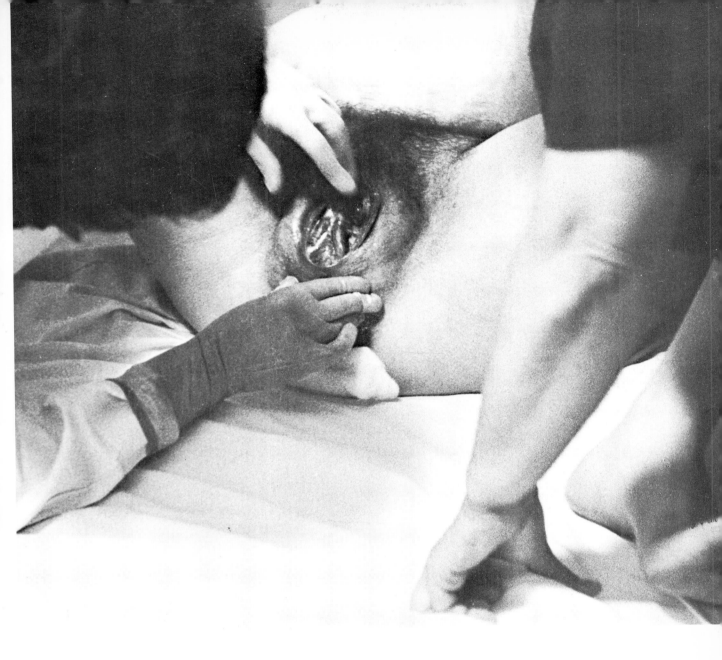

WITH EACH CONTRACTION the head comes down a little farther. At last it is down so far that the mother's whole perineum, the tissue bridge between the back edge of the vagina and the front edge of the anus, bulges.

Here the wrinkles on the baby's scalp can be clearly seen. They are there partly because the baby's head is compressed and partly because of "caput," an accumulation of edema fluid, which collects over whatever part of the baby is born first and is thus under special pressure. The swelling of caput is often visible for some hours after the baby's birth, but it gradually disappears.

In this photograph the doctor's right hand is "guarding" the mother's perineum. He is trying to make sure that it does not tear. The mother is most likely to tear as the head is born, and she is less likely to do so if she can cooperate with her attendants and push harder or not so hard, according to instructions. Tears are commoner with first than with later babies, but some women seem to be so constructed that they tear with every baby, no matter how well they cooperate or how skillful their attendants are.

If the patient is certainly going to tear, or else if the pressure of the mother's muscles is putting a strain on the baby's head, many doctors perform a small operation called an episiotomy. Local anesthetic is injected, and a cut is made in the mother's perineum so that the baby's head can slip through easily. This is sewn up again as soon as the baby is born, before the effects of the local anesthetic have worn off.

In some cultures the whole procedure is entirely different, and the woman is delivered sitting in a chair, standing, squatting, or even tied to a tree.

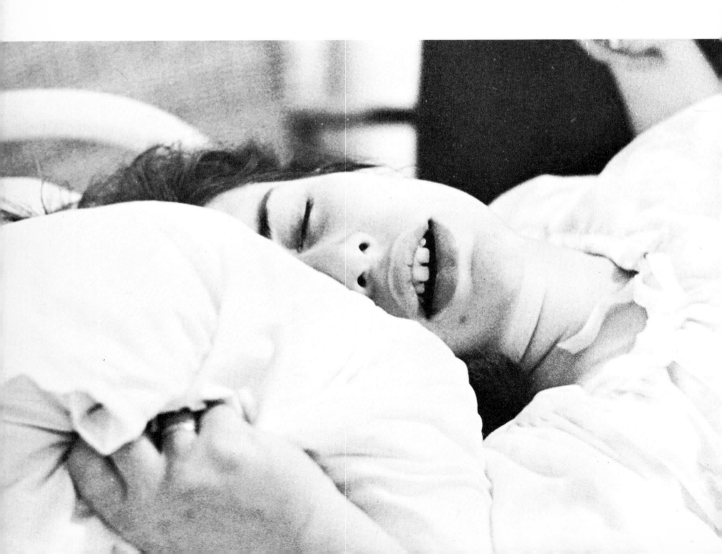

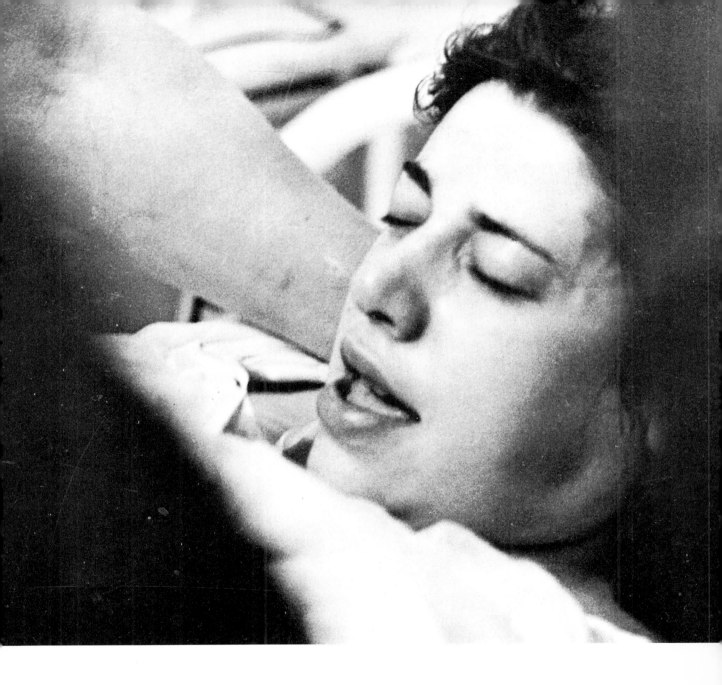

AS SHE PUSHES, an expression of satisfaction comes over the mother's face. She finds that the pain is not nearly so troublesome because she has something to do and can push with it. She is concentrating hard, probably breathing between pushes. It is hard work. But she now has the satisfaction of knowing that soon her baby will be born.

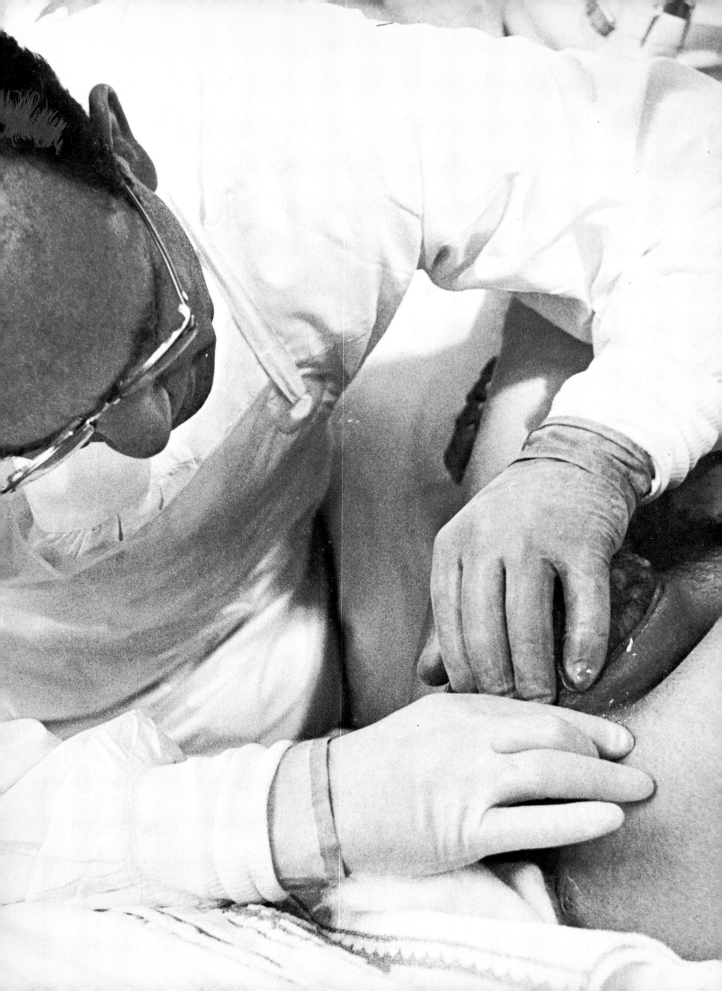

THE HEAD CROWNS. At this stage the mother is asked to stop pushing, though for some this seems an impossible feat since the desire to push is often overwhelming. The doctor is still carefully guarding the perineum with his right hand. With his left hand he is controlling the birth of the baby's head. He is probably trying to make the baby bend its head farther downward toward its chest, because this means that there is a smaller diameter of head to stretch the mother. If the baby's head is flexed and emerges slowly, it is less likely to tear the mother's perineum as it comes through.

WHILE THE MOTHER IS RESTING, the doctor eases the rest of the baby's head and face out of the birth canal.

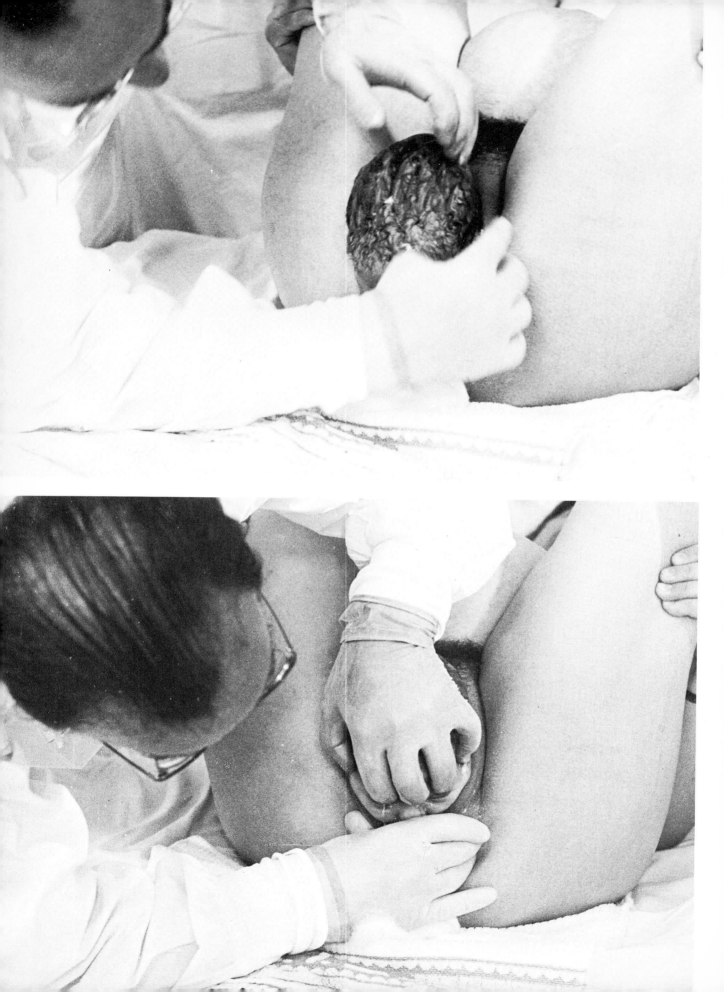

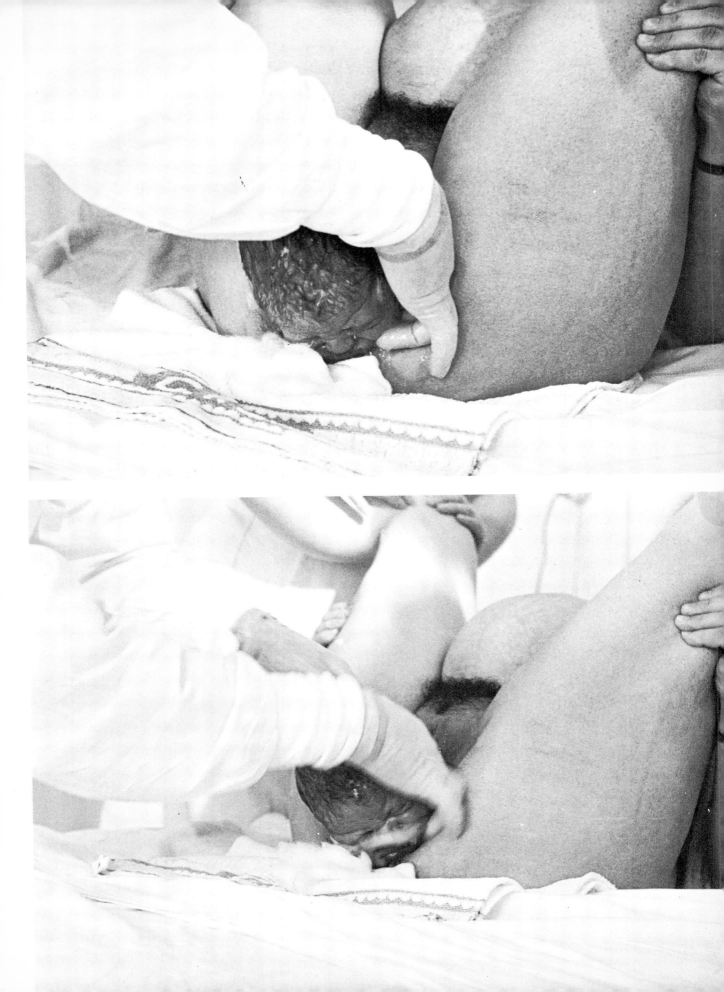

The baby's head is born facing toward the mother's anus. While it is being born, the baby has to pass through the mother's pelvis, a ring of bones that encircles her body and forms a curved tunnel with bony walls. The baby's head is the largest part, and once the head is born the rest of the body will follow. When both baby and mother are of normal size, the head of the baby is a tight fit in the mother's pelvis. To some extent this is overcome by "molding," a process in which the soft bones of the baby's skull gradually take up the shape and diameter of the mother's pelvis.

The bony tunnel of the mother's pelvis is not the same shape all the way down. For this reason the baby makes various turns of its head and body to negotiate the canal in the easiest possible way. As the baby's head enters the pelvis, it has to turn to fit itself to the shape of the mother; and so lies slightly sideways. The baby's head often goes down into the pelvis some days or weeks before labor starts, particularly in a first pregnancy. When this happens the mother may feel more comfortable, and this is known as "lightening." The baby's head now lies deep in the pelvis, and so there is more room to accommodate the rest of the baby. It does not come up so high under her ribs or feel so heavy and ungainly, but in many cases, most often in women who have had babies before, the head does not enter the pelvis until labor has started.

For the mother the birth of the baby's head is one of the most difficult parts of labor, and at this stage she is particularly likely to lose control. She feels a host of new and powerful sensations which she may not understand, recognize, or be able to deal with. The descent of the baby's head is unlike anything else that ever happened to her, and it produces its own unique reactions. She may feel intensely excited, disturbed, frightened, or ecstatic. She may feel that she is "splitting in two" or she may be conscious of no more than a strong desire to pass a large stool. Women vary very much in their sensations and also in the time it takes for the baby's head to pass through the birth canal.

The birth of the baby's head is one of the events of labor for which proper training during pregnancy is most useful. Childbirth classes are now held in many hospitals and clinics; others are organized by an obstetrician for his own patients, by visiting nurse associations, or by the Red Cross. Mothers are taught what to expect, how to deal with the various sensations that they will feel, and how to enjoy the whole business of producing a baby.

As soon as the baby's head is born, it begins to turn. This is because the head became slightly twisted on the shoulders in order to negotiate the bony tunnel and it is now righting itself. The shoulders are still inside the mother and slightly turned toward her left side. The baby is straightening its head in relation to its own shoulders.

This baby is being born in one of the commonest positions and one likely to go with the easiest birth. In this position the smallest diameter of the baby's head can most easily pass through the birth canal, and so an easy passage is likely.

The shoulders are now descending through the birth passage, and as they do this they turn still further until they are at right angles to the mother. In this way they take up what is the easiest position for them. Thus, for the rest of the birth, the baby is facing sideways.

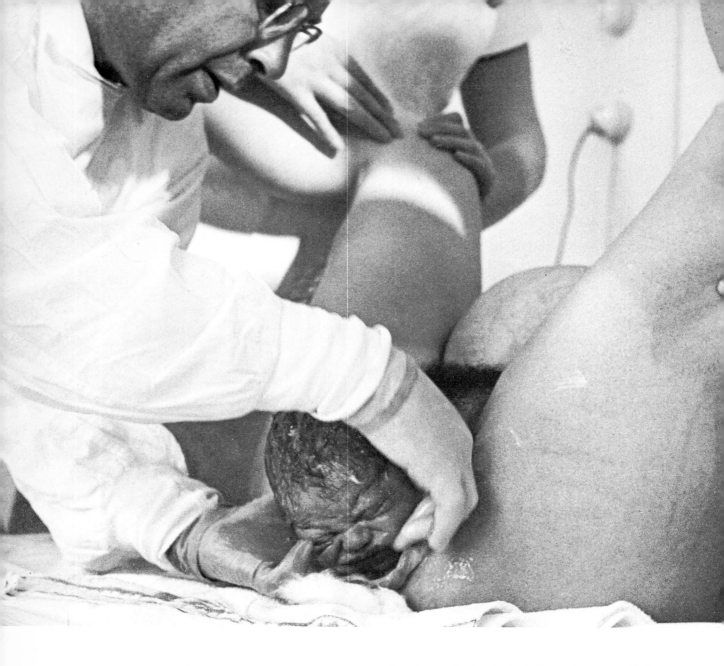

As soon as the head is born, the doctor feels the baby's neck to see if the umbilical cord is wound round it. Usually it is not, but it happens often enough to make this one of the important duties of whoever delivers the baby. If the cord is present but very loose, it is possible to slip it over the baby's head and out of the way. If it is fairly loose, it can be eased gently to the side and the rest of the baby can be delivered through the loop. If the cord is wound very tightly round the baby's neck, neither of these two procedures is possible and the doctor then puts two clamps on the cord, to prevent bleeding, cuts between the clamps and unwinds the cord. This frees the baby and enables its body to be born.

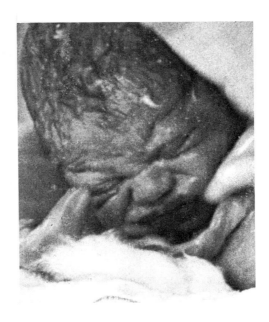

IN THIS CASE the doctor finds that the cord is round the baby's neck, but only loosely. He knows he will be able to deliver the rest of the baby through the loop.

The umbilical cord is usually about 20 inches long, and it runs from the navel of the baby to the center (occasionally to the side) of the placenta.

It may be half an inch or less in thickness or more than an inch. It gives the appearance of being twisted because the vessels inside it run a spiral course. Most of the thickness is made up of a jelly-like substance, called Wharton's jelly, which cushions and protects the three blood vessels that run in it—two umbilical arteries and one umbilical vein.

These are the blood vessels that are part of the baby's circulation, with the umbilical vein carrying red blood full of oxygen and nourishment and the two umbilical arteries carrying the baby's blood which has lost most of its oxygen and nutriments and contains waste products to be disposed of.

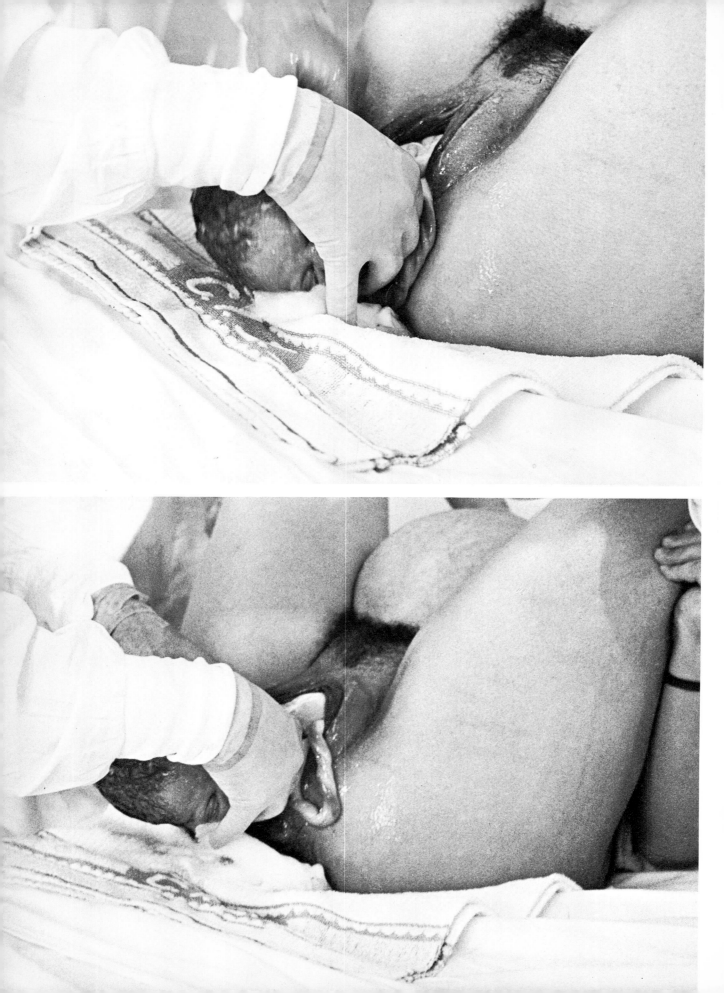

WHEN THE BABY'S HEAD has turned itself completely sideways, the shoulders are ready to be born. The first shoulder appears and can be seen just above the doctor's knuckle in these pictures. The doctor bends the baby's head and neck gently downward toward the bed to help the birth of the "anterior shoulder." This is the shoulder lying to the front of the mother, in this case the baby's left shoulder; the baby's front shoulder is usually delivered first. It shows up white because it is covered with *vernix caseosa,* a greasy material mainly manufactured by the baby's own oil glands in the skin. It probably helps to protect the baby's skin. The cord has been pushed to one side, well out of the way.

As soon as the first shoulder is born, the doctor bends the baby's head and neck upward toward the mother's front. This helps the birth of the back shoulder, the one lying nearest the bed.

This baby looks rather blue (compare its color with that of the mother and her attendants). He has been deprived of oxygen for the last few minutes while his body was descending through the birth canal. But there is no cause for alarm. Luckily a baby, unlike older children and adults, has tremendous powers of withstanding relatively long periods without oxygen. As long as he breathes fairly soon, no harm will result.

ONCE THE HEAD AND SHOULDERS ARE BORN, the rest is easy. The baby's body and legs slip out without trouble.

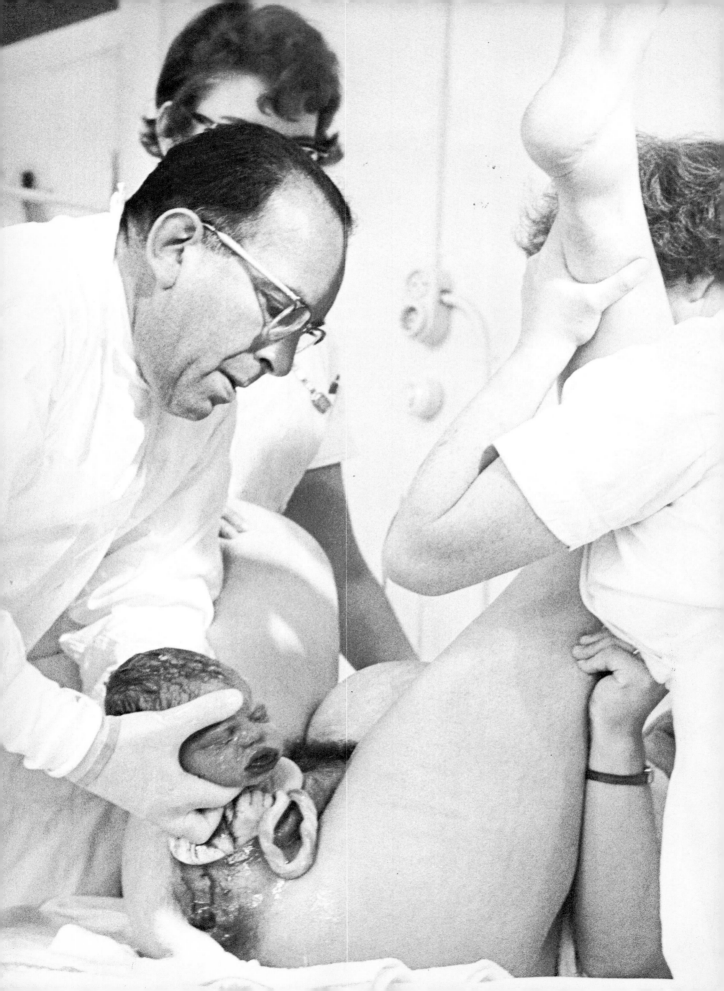

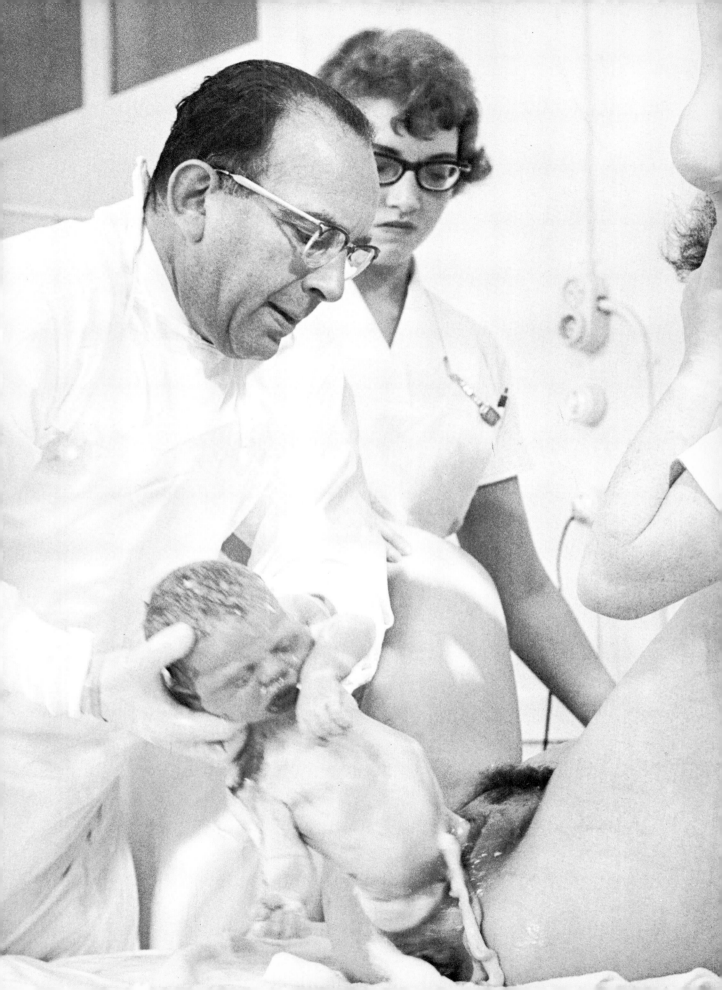

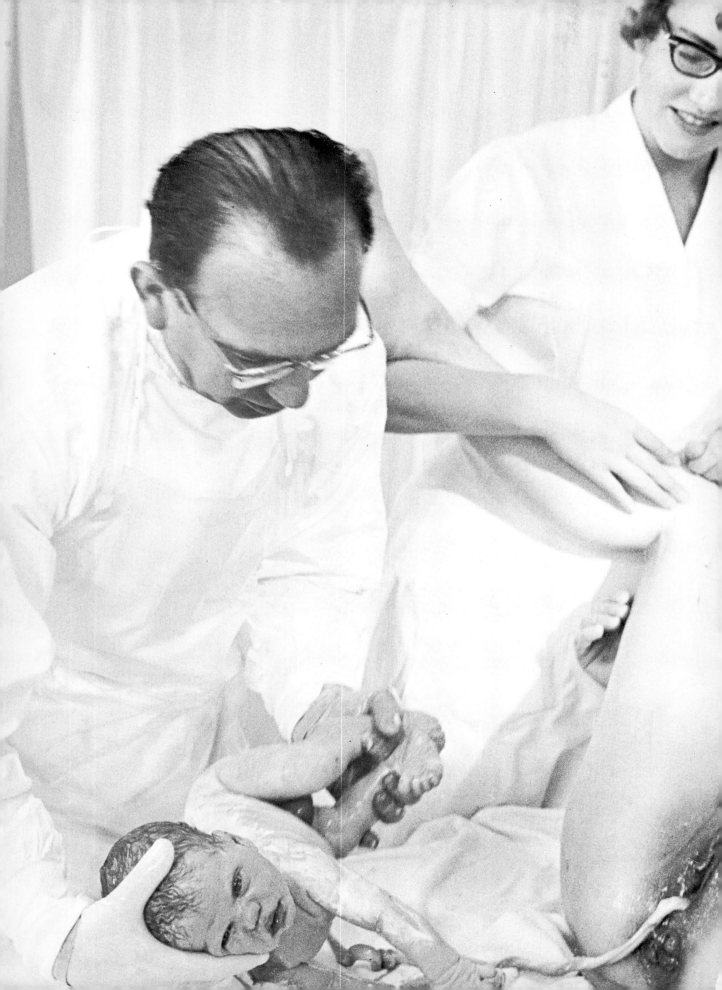

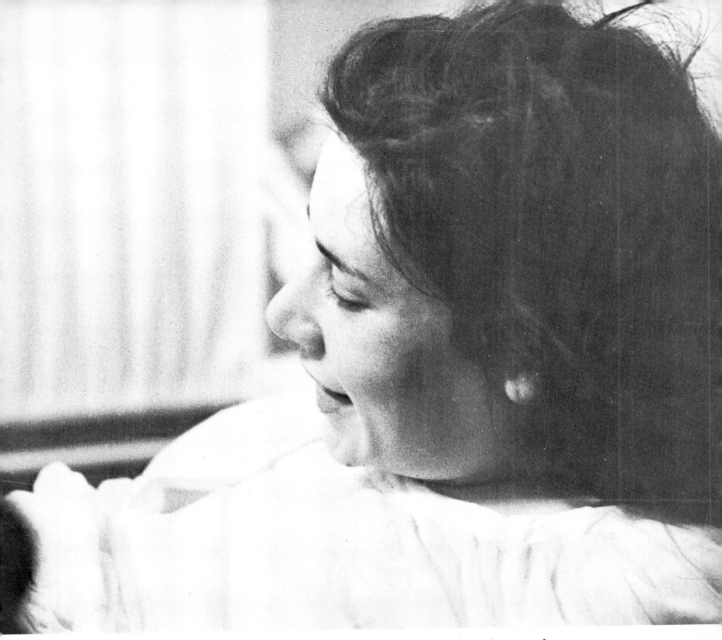

IT'S A BOY! The mother catches a first glimpse of her child before he disappears from view again.

THE DOCTOR HAS the whole baby in his hands. Still very blue, he has not yet cried or breathed, but he has already opened his eyes and will breathe at any moment. He is still attached to his mother by his cord, and is covered by *vernix caseosa.*

THE DOCTOR HOLDS HIM upside down to let any liquid that he may have breathed in run out. He takes a gauze swab and wipes out the baby's mouth. If the mother is watching, she may be struck by the large size and deep blue color of his scrotum, but this is normal.

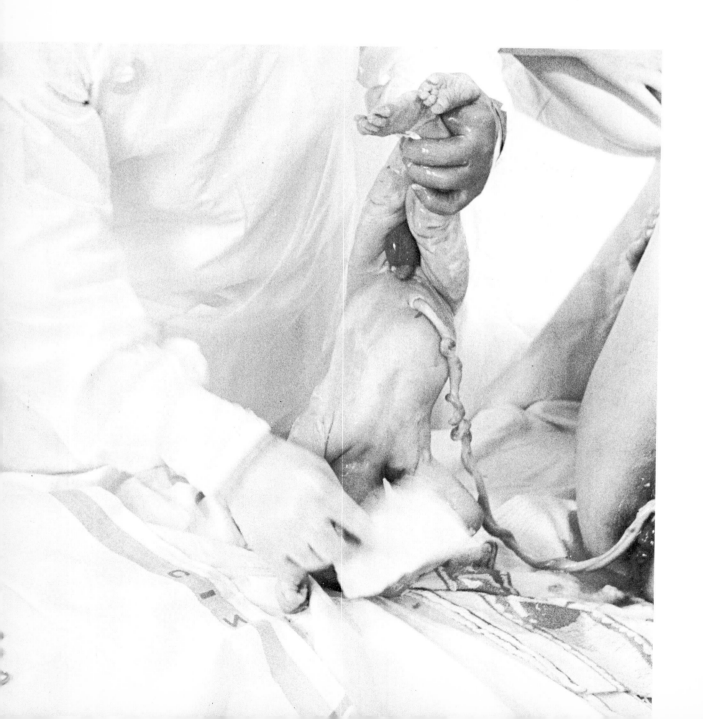

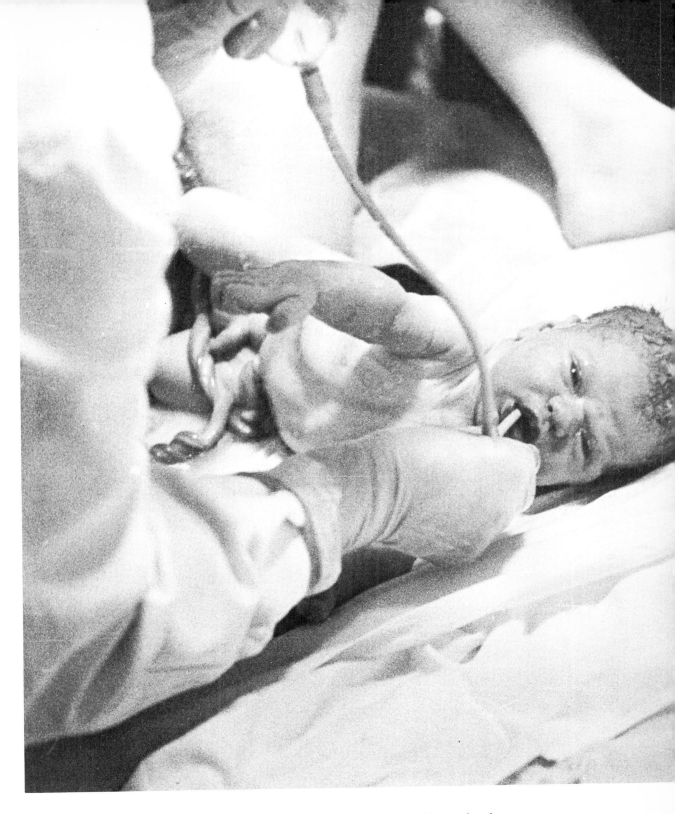

THE DOCTOR SUCKS OUT the baby's mouth and throat with a rubber tube, because it is important to clear the airway. If it is blocked the baby will not be able to breathe, or will inhale liquid and other stuff into his lungs.

THE DOCTOR HOLDS the baby upside down again and rocks and pats him gently to stimulate breathing. The nurse talks encouragingly to the mother, who may be worried because her baby has not yet cried.

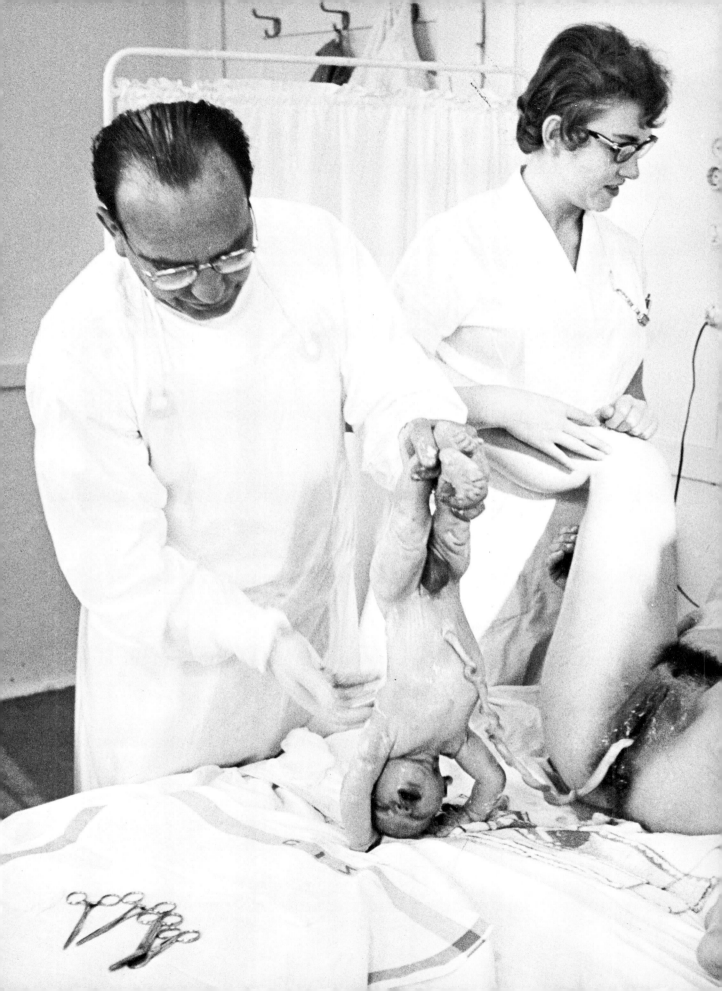

THE DOCTOR DECIDES that the moment has come to separate the baby from his mother. He doubly clamps the cord so that it will not bleed from either end when it is cut.

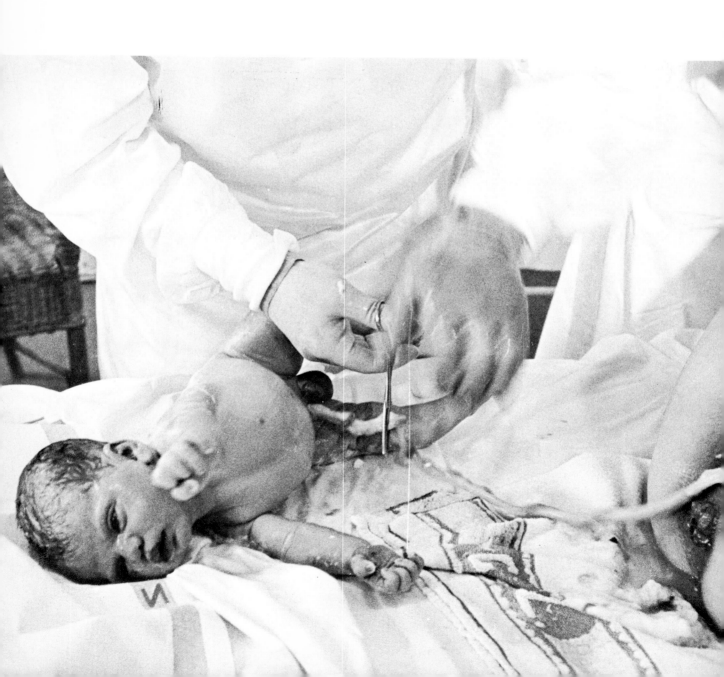

THEN HE TAKES a pair of scissors and cuts the cord. There is no sensation in the cord, so the baby feels nothing.

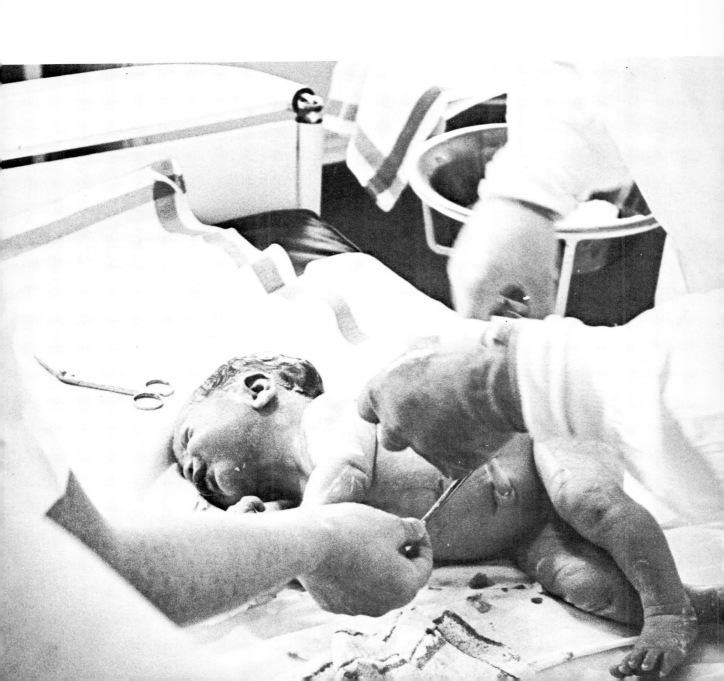

THE BABY, suddenly separated from his mother, takes his first breath, and yells furiously. With his first few breaths his deep blue color, which can be most alarming to the untrained observer, changes to a healthy pink. Many babies breathe as soon as they are born, before the cord is cut.

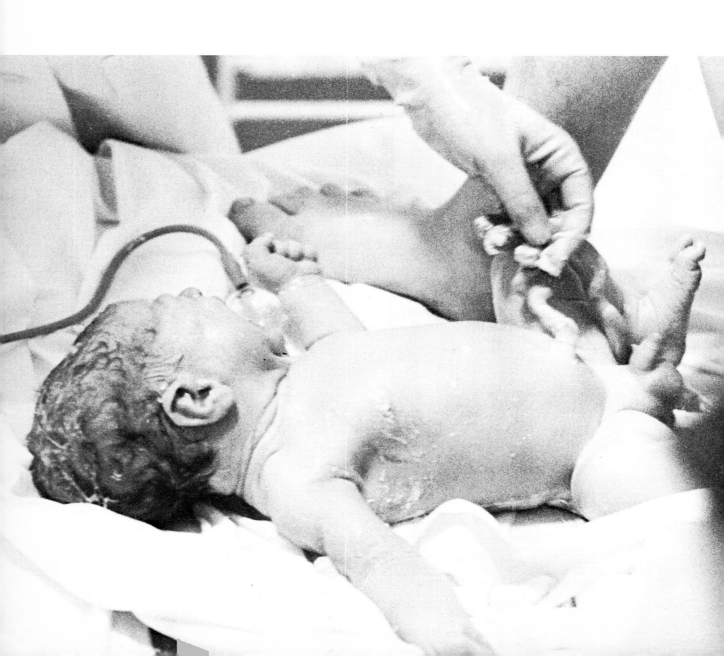

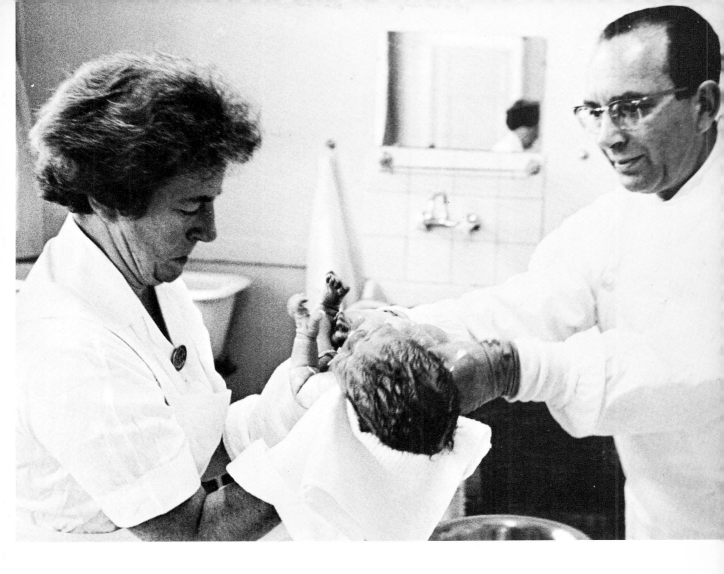

THE NURSE WRAPS the baby in a warmed blanket. Exhausted with the whole business of being born and yelling afterward, he falls asleep. At this stage he may be given to his mother. He may even suck at her breast, and some nurses and doctors like the baby to suck at this early stage because the sucking instinct is strongest at birth. There is also a nervous reflex by which the baby's sucking causes the womb to contract, and this helps the afterbirth to be born and reduces the danger of bleeding. The same reflex can also cause the "afterpains" the mother may feel in her stomach during the few days following the birth. These are liable to be particularly strong while she is feeding the baby. In this way the baby helps his mother, first of all with the last stage of her labor and later in restoring her womb to its normal condition.

AT THIS STAGE the mother probably feels that all is over, but the doctor knows that it is not. The mother still has to go through the third stage of labor, in which the afterbirth is born. During this final stage she needs careful supervision to make sure that all is well. The doctor now hands the baby over to the nurse and turns back to his patient. He has to make sure that the afterbirth comes away properly, completely, and without excessive bleeding. He watches the mother carefully, and she probably feels no pain. If the perineum has torn, the doctor will stitch it, probably under local anesthesia.

THE AFTERBIRTH may be born almost immediately or not for twenty minutes or more. But until it is safely delivered there is always the danger of bleeding, so that if it does not arrive within an hour or so the mother will be given an anesthetic and the doctor will remove the afterbirth with his hand.

As long as the placenta or afterbirth is inside her, the mother is still in labor. The placenta, attached to the inside wall of her womb, develops with the baby.

Soon after the baby is born, the placenta separates itself from the wall of the uterus. Attached to it are the membranes that surrounded the baby when he was inside. These formed the bag of waters.

THE DOCTOR examines it carefully to make sure that none of it has been left inside. He is holding the membranes and displaying the baby's side of the placenta. The blood vessels gathering themselves into the umbilical cord can be seen clearly. The doctor is holding the cut end of the umbilical cord with his right hand, and the other end of the cord can be seen where it disappears into the afterbirth.

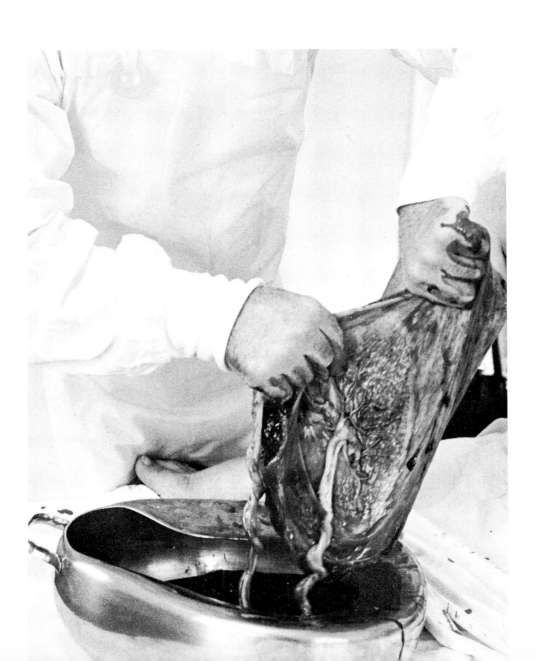

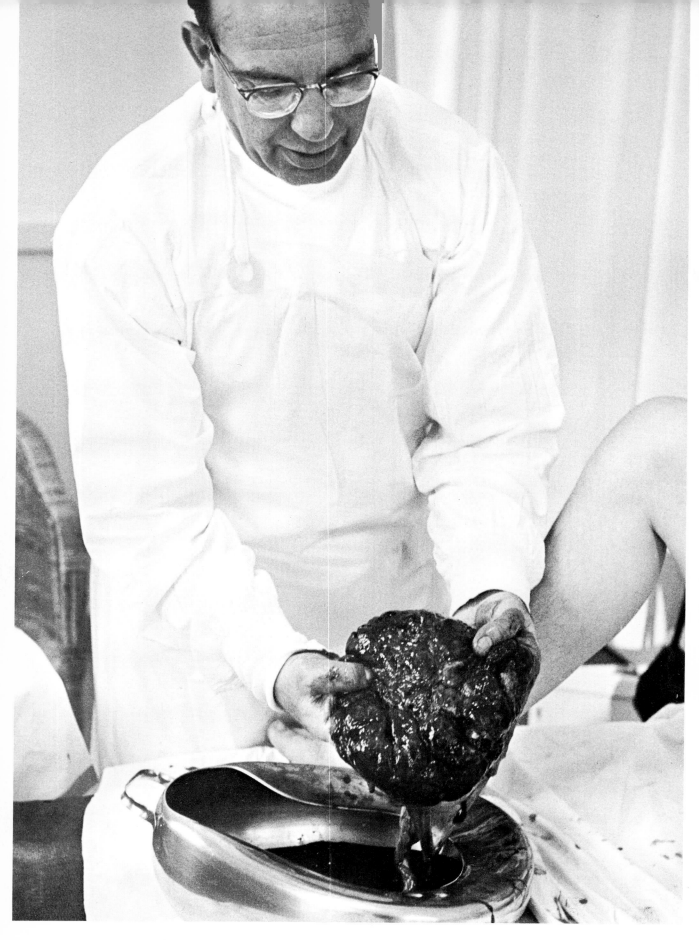

THIS IS THE RAW SIDE of the placenta, which, until a few seconds ago, was attached to the wall of the mother's womb. This is where the mother's blood flowed and where the food, oxygen, and other products that it carried diffused through the afterbirth and flowed into the baby.

The doctor decides that the placenta is complete and that all is well. If by any chance he discovered that part of it was missing, he would give the mother a light anesthetic and recover the missing piece with his finger.

THE BABY IS WEIGHED, washed and dressed . . .

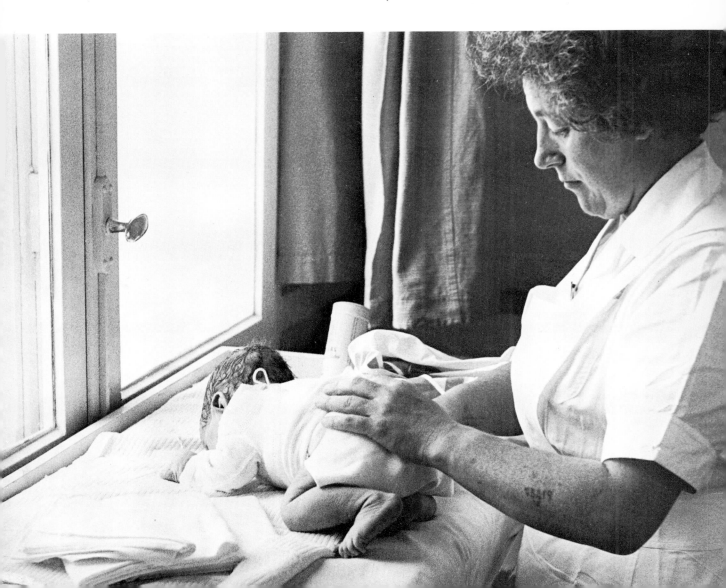

. . . and handed to his mother.

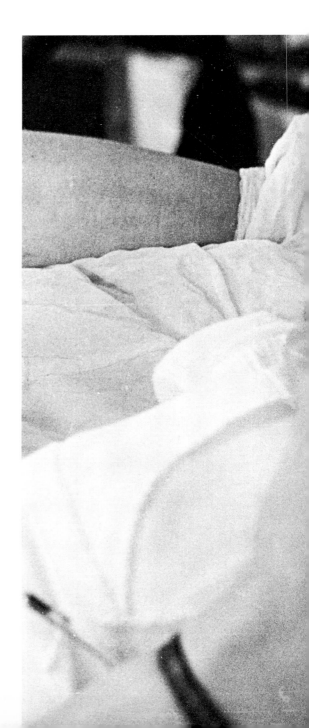

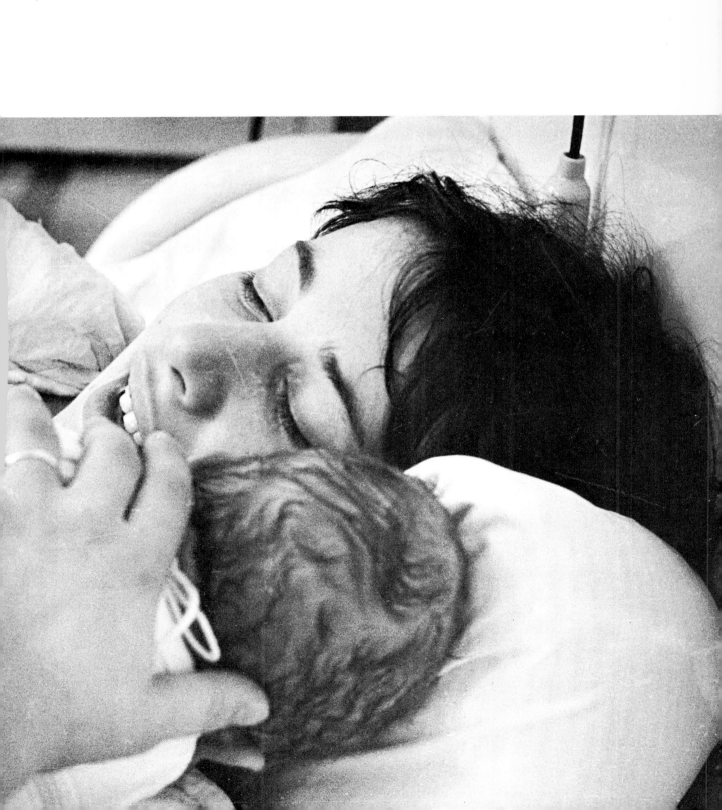

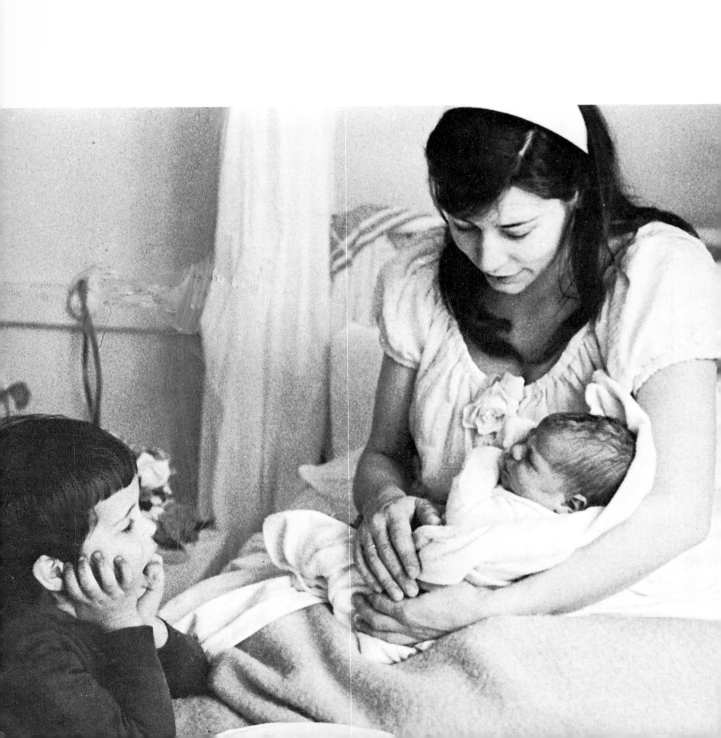